HATHAYOGA

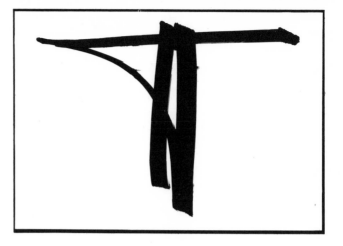

WALTER AMES COMPTON

STEVEN KATONA,
PHOTOGRAPHS

HARPER COLOPHON BOOKS   HARPER & ROW, PUBLISHERS
NEW YORK   EVANSTON   SAN FRANCISCO   LONDON

HATHAYOGA. PHOTOGRAPHS & TEXT COPYRIGHT © 1974 BY *WALTER A. COMPTON*.
ALL RIGHTS RESERVED. PRINTED IN THE UNITED STATES OF AMERICA. NO PART
OF THIS BOOK MAY BE USED OR REPRODUCED IN ANY MANNER WITHOUT WRITTEN
PERMISSION EXCEPT IN THE CASE OF BRIEF QUOTATIONS EMBODIED IN CRITICAL
ARTICLES AND REVIEWS. FOR INFORMATION ADDRESS *HARPER & ROW, PUBLISHERS,
INC.*, 10 EAST 53RD STREET, NEW YORK, N.Y. 10022. PUBLISHED SIMULTANEOUSLY
IN CANADA BY *FITZHENRY & WHITESIDE LIMITED*, TORONTO.

FIRST *HARPER COLOPHON* EDITION PUBLISHED 1974

LIBRARY OF CONGRESS CATALOGUE CARD NUMBER: 74-3520

STANDARD BOOK NUMBER: 06-090379-1

HATHA, SANSKRIT FOR VIOLENCE, AND *YOGA*

A YOKING

IS ALSO *HA* THE SUN, *THA* MOON, AND *YOGA*

THEIR CLEAR FUSION INTO LIGHT AND DARK

OF PLACE.

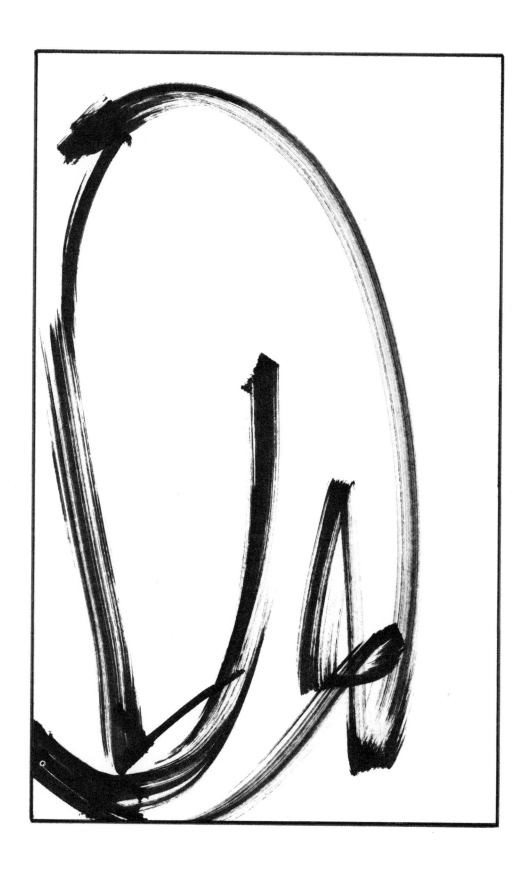

HATHAYOGA
MEDITATION

SHRIVEL THE COLD TWISTING

MIND, AS YOU

THRASH YOURSELF INTO CRACKING AIR.

BE STILL.

SPIN LUMINOUS BREATH ABOUT YOUR PAIN.

SOOTHE IT INTO A CENTER.

CONTAIN IT IN PLACING HANDS.

MEDITATION IS A HEALING.

MEDITATION IS DESPAIR.

CRY THE FLIGHT OF YOUR ILLUSIONS TO THEIR

ULTIMATE ABSURDITY.

RAGE BEYOND RAGE.

THEN QUIETLY,

    DESPAIR OF YOUR DESPAIR.

RETURN.

MEDITATION IS HATHAYOGA.

BREATH INTO BREATH,
BREATHE YOUR MIND CLEAR.

BALANCING ARM AGAINST ARM, LEG AGAINST LEG,
DRAW SMOOTH AIR
THROUGH THE NOSE, DOWN INTO THE LUNGS AND INTO
FULL ARTICULATE INWARD AND OUTWARD EXTENSION OF
BONE, JOINT, AND MUSCLE
AS SELF.

A SINGLE BREATH BEGINS LIFE.
IT ALSO BEGINS AND SUSTAINS HATHAYOGA.
EVOLVING *ĀSANA*, THE SEATS OF POSITION, IN THE
SINGING RESONANCE OF *PRĀṆA*, UNIVERSAL VIBRATION,
BREATH LIFTS YOU ON POINTED STILLNESS
INTO THE CENTER OF
WHERE YOU ARE.

PADMĀSANA:
LOTUS POSE

WITH LEGS CROSSED ONE ABOVE THE OTHER,
LOCKING INTO A FIRM LEVEL SEAT,
CENTER THE HANDS IN YOGA MUDRĀ,
THE GESTURE OF YOGA.

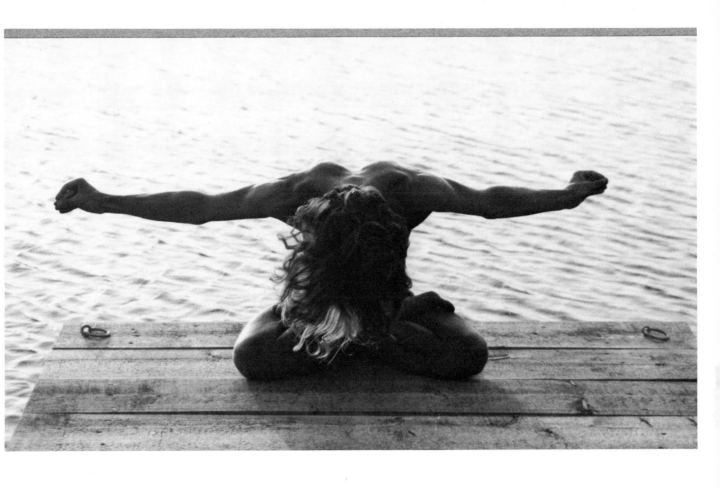

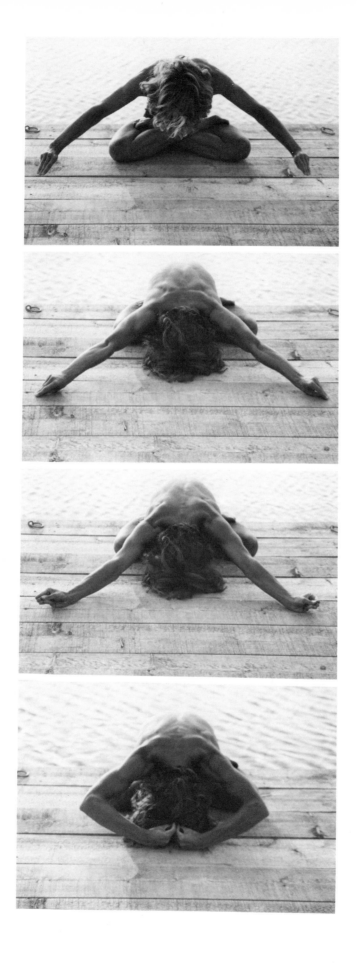

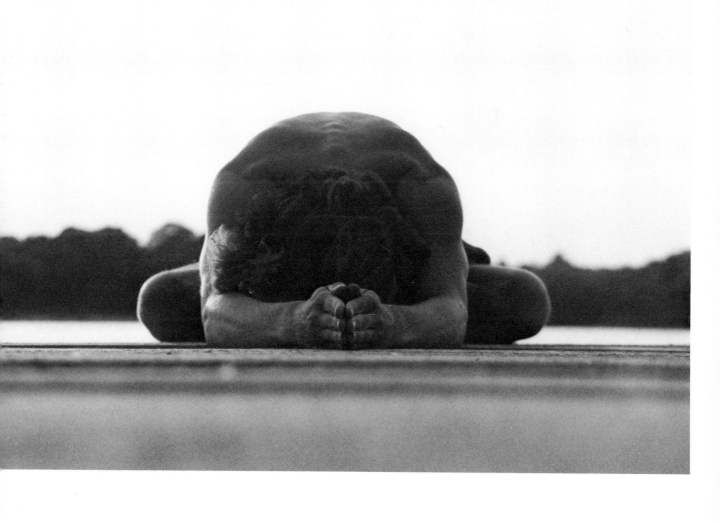

CRADLE SOFTLY INTO SPINNING EASE

RELEASE

RETURN

RISE UP INTO YOUR BREATH

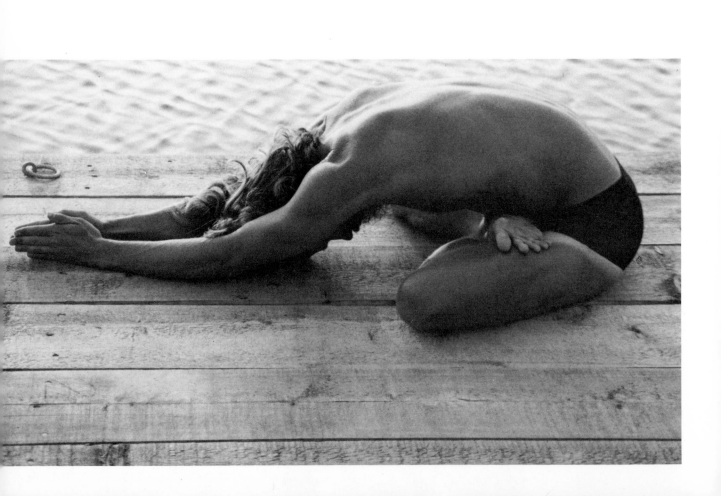

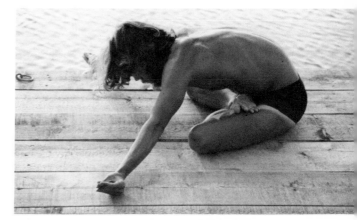

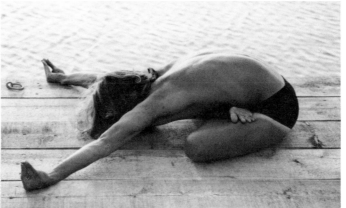

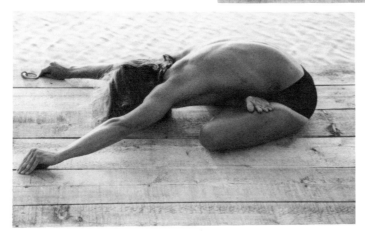

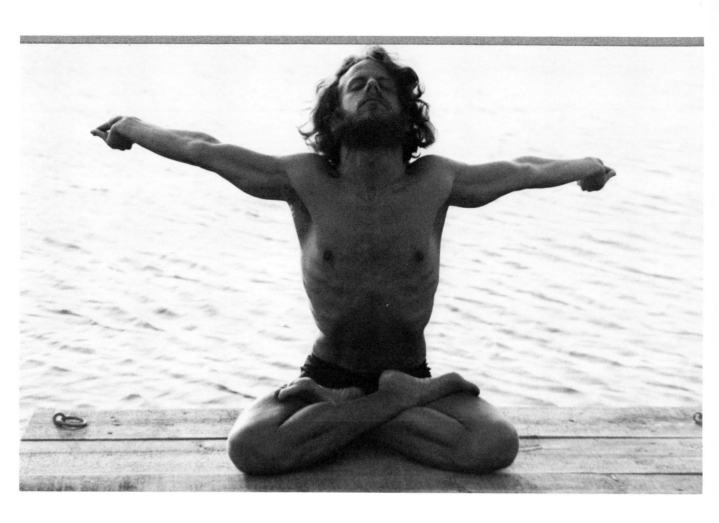

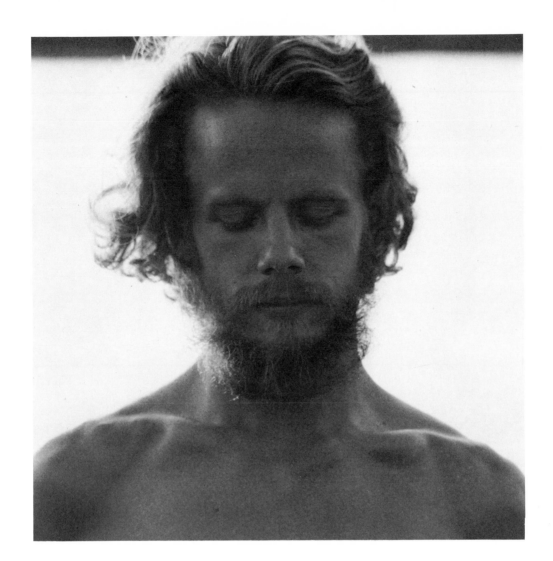

ARDHA PADMOTTĀNĀSANA:
HALF EXTENDED-LOTUS POSE

STANDING INTO A SINGLE FOOT,
BEND FORWARD,
CLOSED.

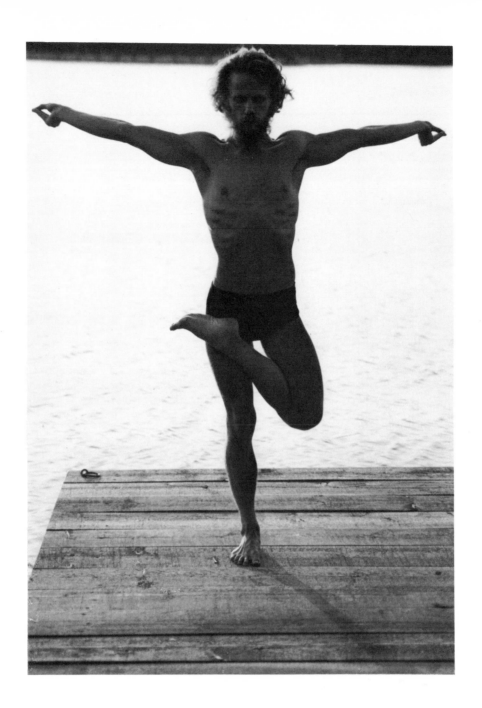

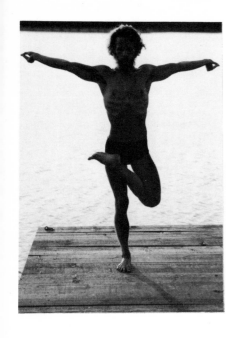
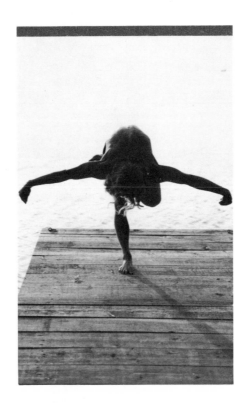

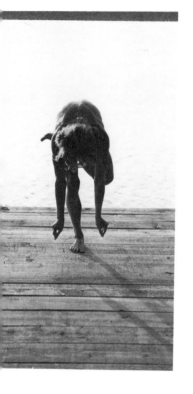
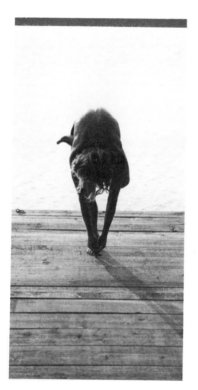
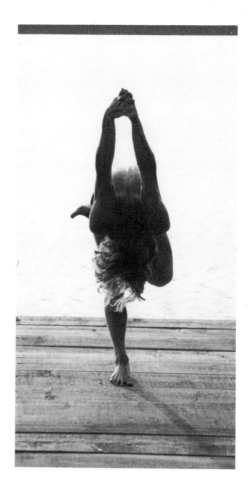

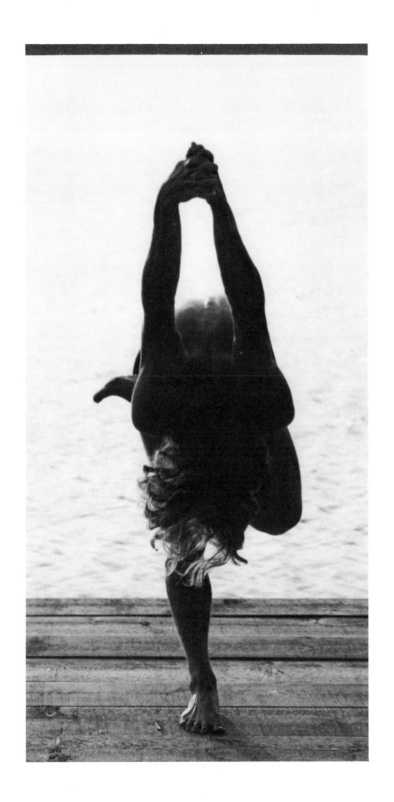

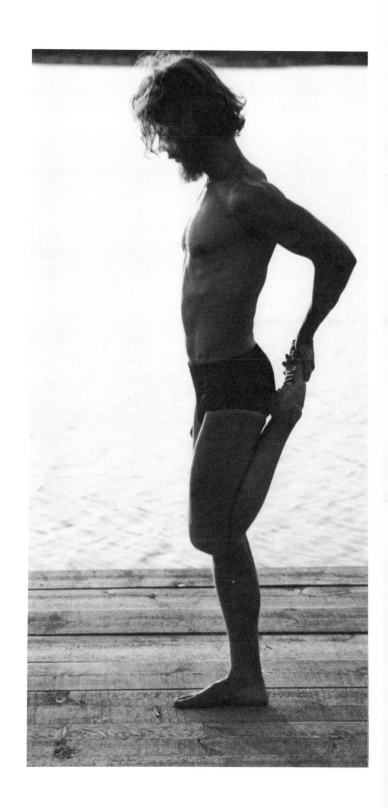

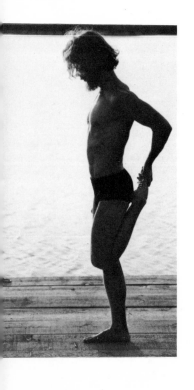

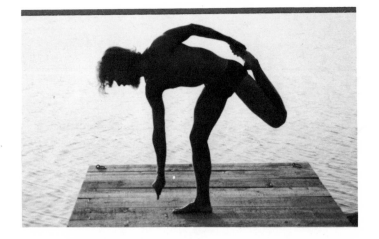

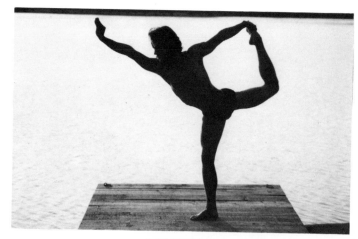

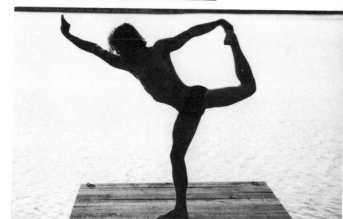

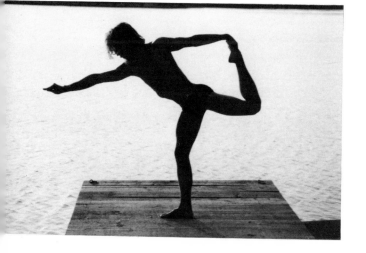

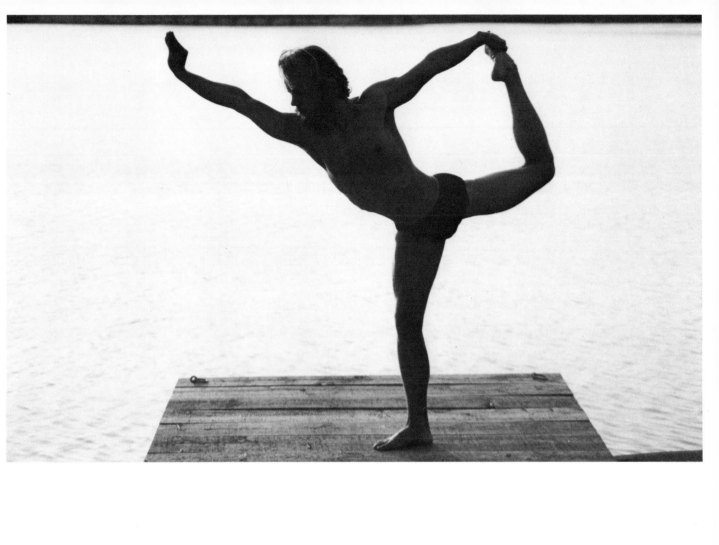

ARDHA ANJANYĀSANA: HALF LEG-DIVIDE POSE

KNEELING INTO A SINGLE LEG,
TURN QUIETLY,
BACKWARD.

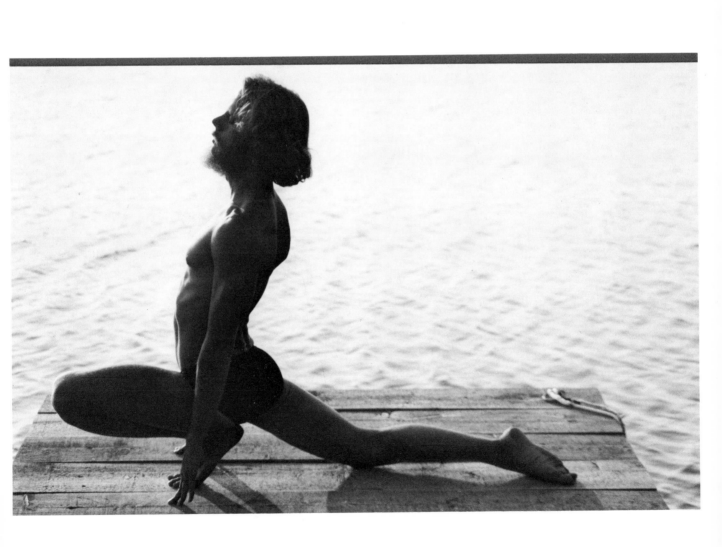

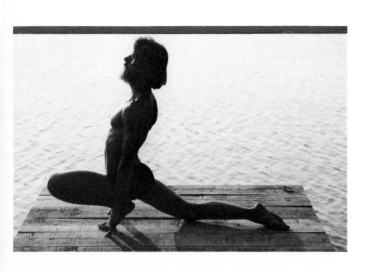

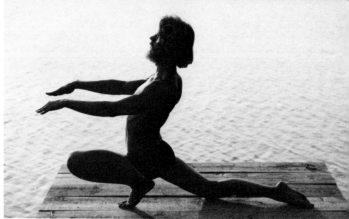

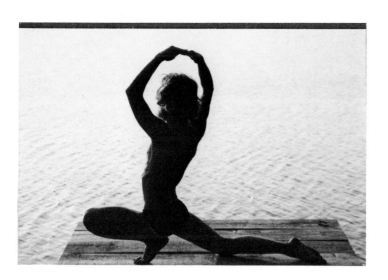
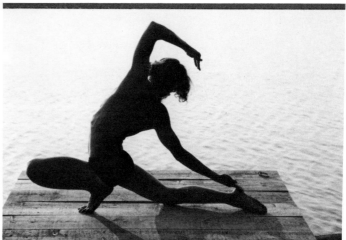

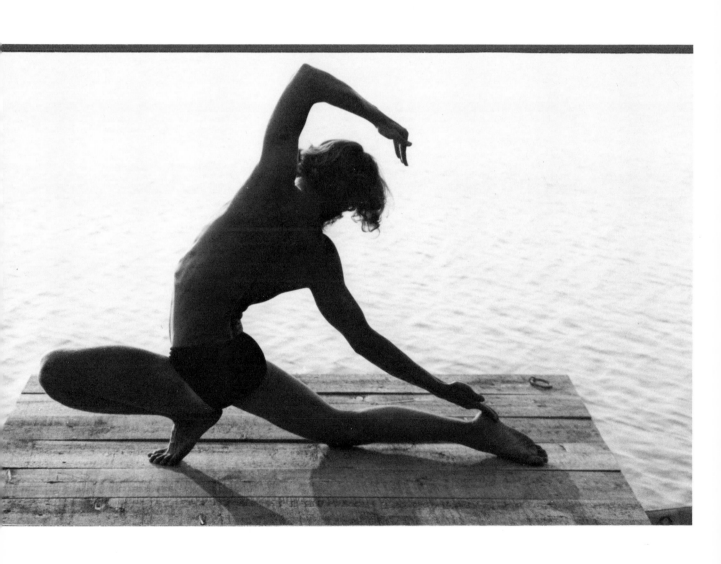

PŪRNA SUPTA-VAJRĀSANA:
DIAMOND FULL-KNEELING POSE

THE SMALL OF THE BACK CARRIES
INTO AN ARCH
THE SWINGING WEIGHT OF TORSO,
HEAD, AND ARMS.

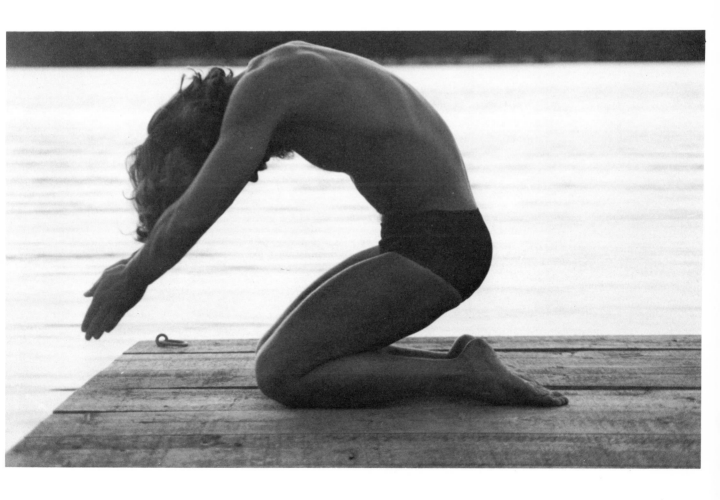

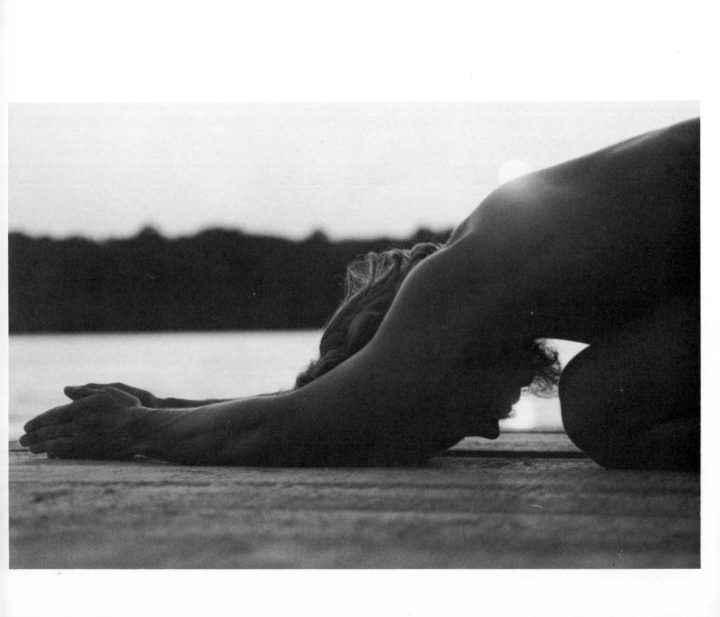

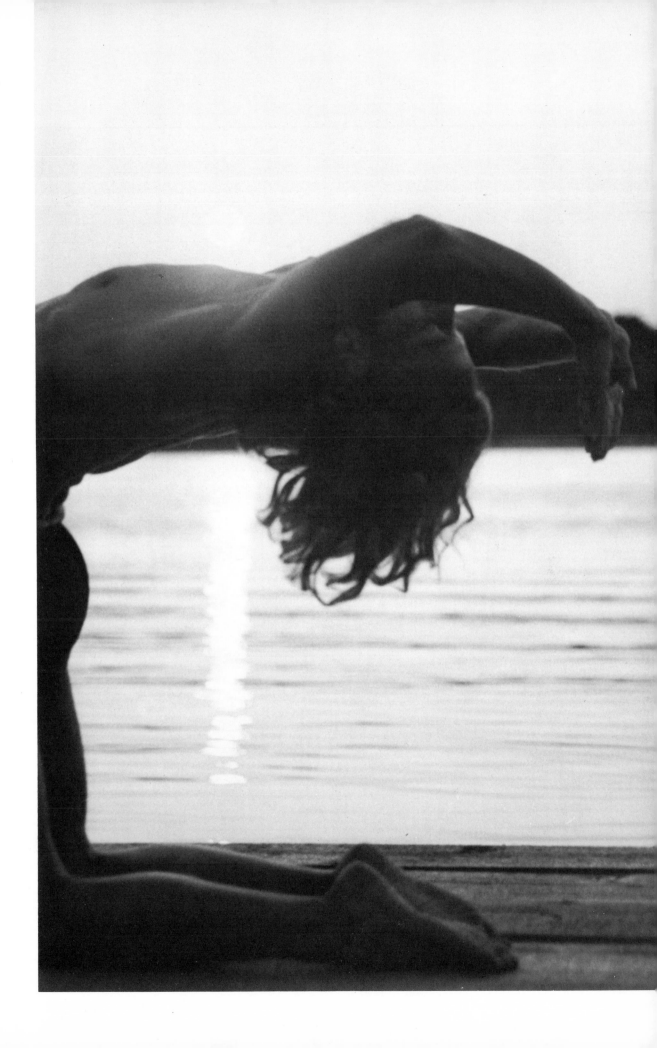

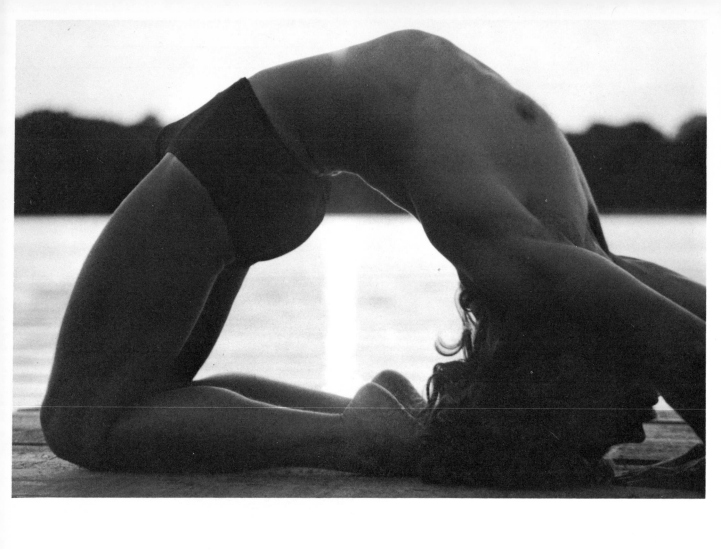

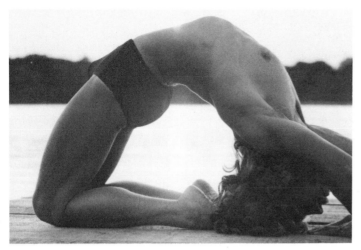

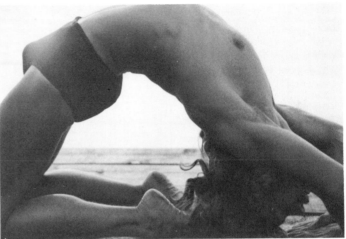

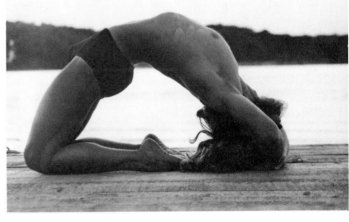

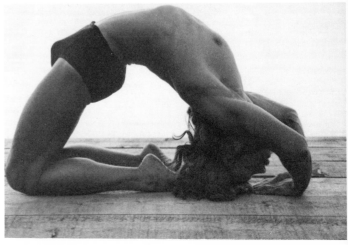

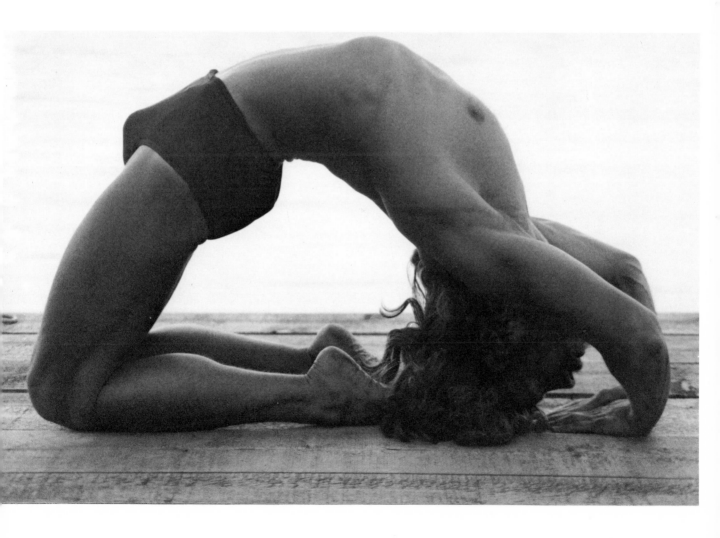

VRỊ̄SCIKĀSANA:
SCORPION POSE

THE SMALL OF THE BACK CARRIES
INTO AN ARCHED CANOPY
LEGS INVERTED IN *SIRSHĀSANA,*
HEADSTAND.

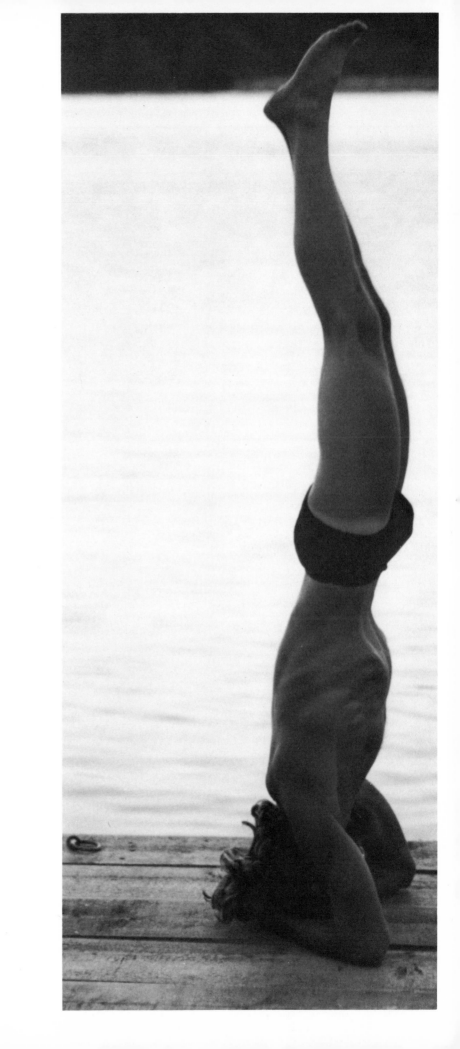

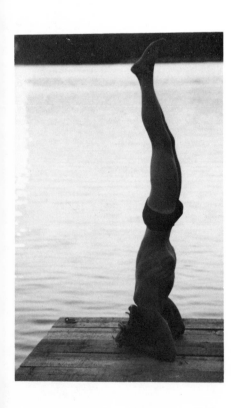
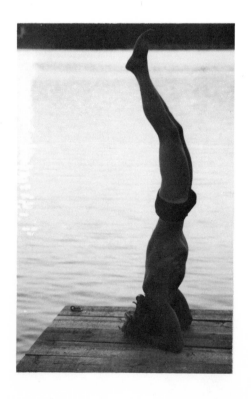

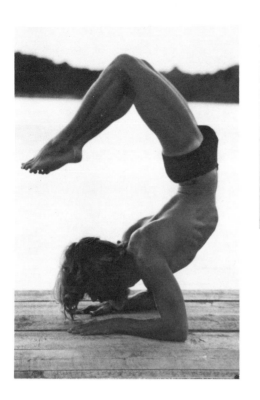

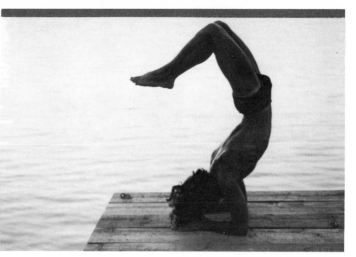

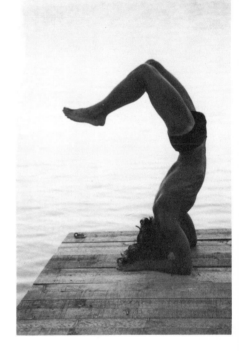

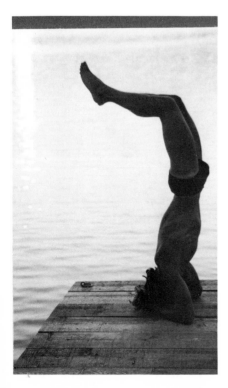

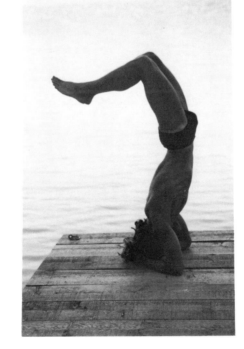

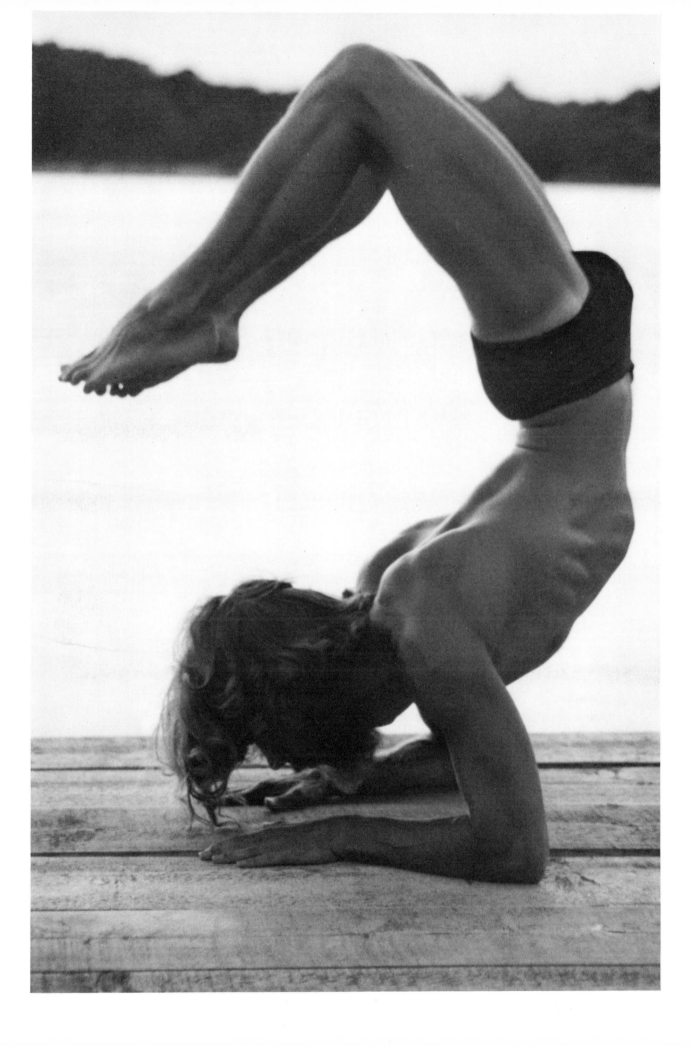

PASHIMOTTĀNĀSANA:
EXTENDED POSTERIOR POSE

THE BODY COUNTERBALANCES ITSELF
INTO AN EASING FORWARD BEND.

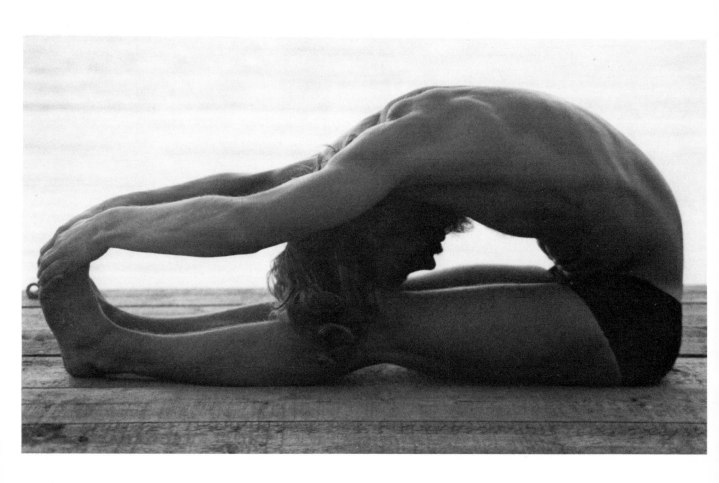

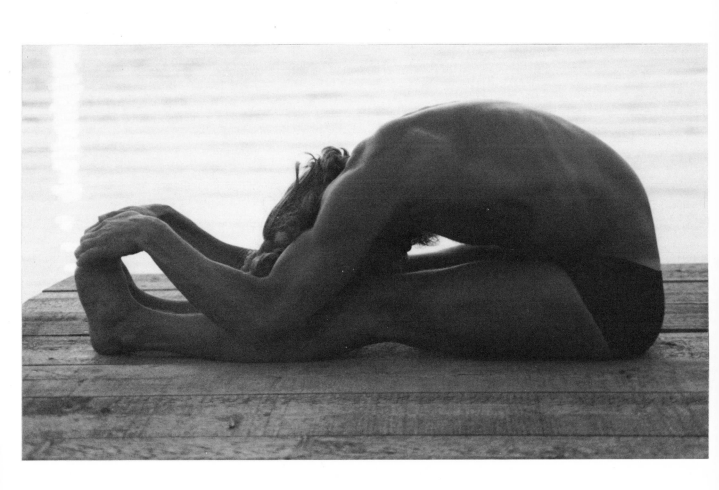

PRĀṆĀYĀMA:
MEDITATION OF BREATH

BEGINNING WITH A RHYTHMIC ALTERNATION
BETWEEN THE BELLOWS DIAPHRAGMATIC BREATH
OF *BASTRIKA,* AND THE REFLEXIVE BREATH
OF *KAPĀLABHĀTI,* AND THEN ENDING WITH LONG
SMOOTH EVEN STROKES, THE LUNGS BRING
VITAL ENERGY INTO THEIR DEPTH,
RETAIN IT THERE,
AND THEN GRADUALLY FILL, STEP BY STEP,
THEIR UPPER PART WHILE HANDS INDICATE
THE *CAKRA* NERVE CENTERS:

> *MŪLĀDHĀRA,* AT THE BASE OF THE SPINAL COLUMN,
> *SVĀDHIṢṬHĀNA,* JUST ABOVE THE GENITALS,
> *MANIPŪRA,* AT THE NAVEL,
> *ANĀHATA,* AT THE CHEST,
> *VISUDDHA,* AT THE THROAT,
> *ĀJÑĀ,* BETWEEN THE EYES,
> > AND
> *SAHASRĀRA,* AT THE CROWN OF THE HEAD.

ARMS FINALLY REACH UPWARD, INDICATING
THE OPEN AND CLOSED COUNTERBALANCES OF
MEDITATION BROUGHT INTO UNION.

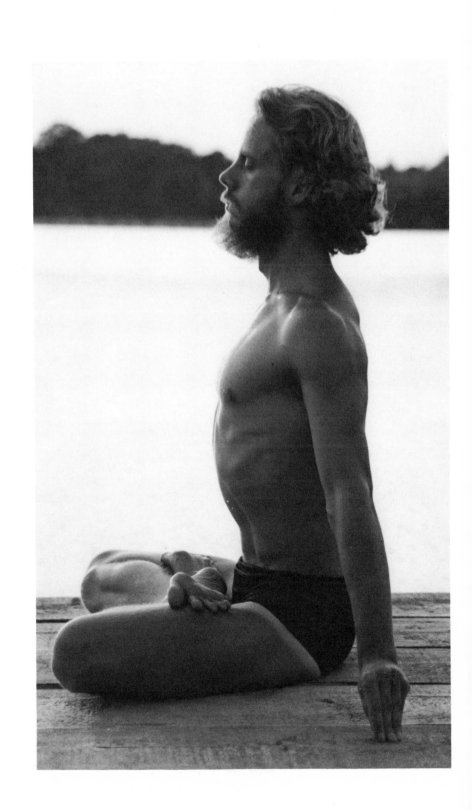

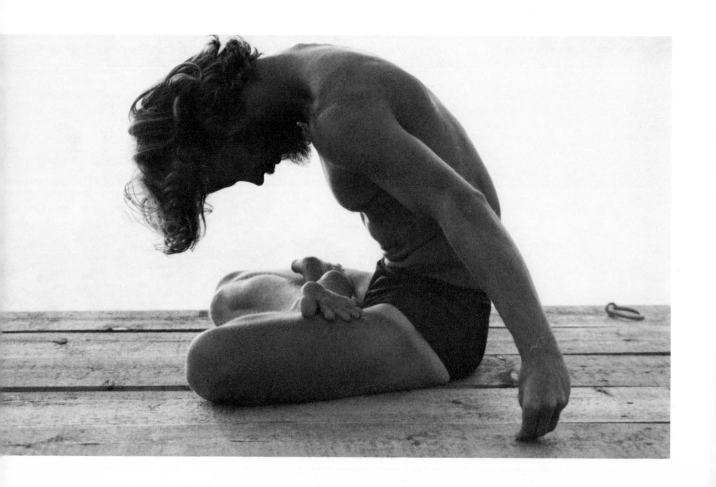

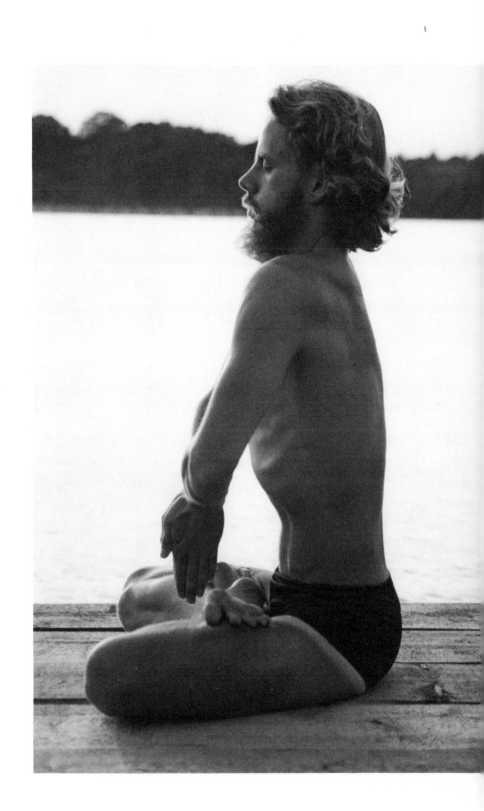

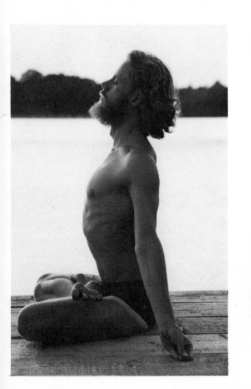

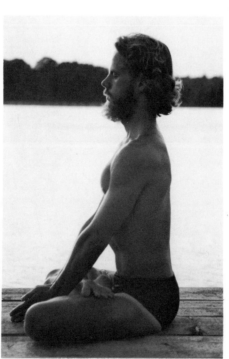

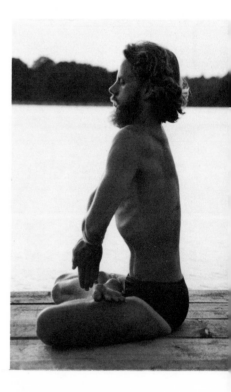

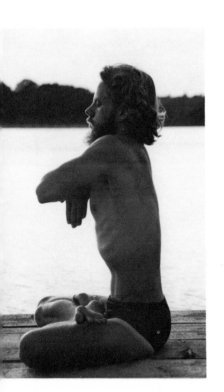
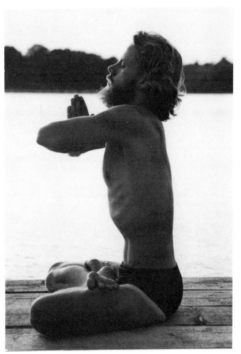
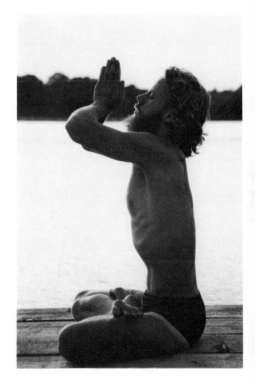

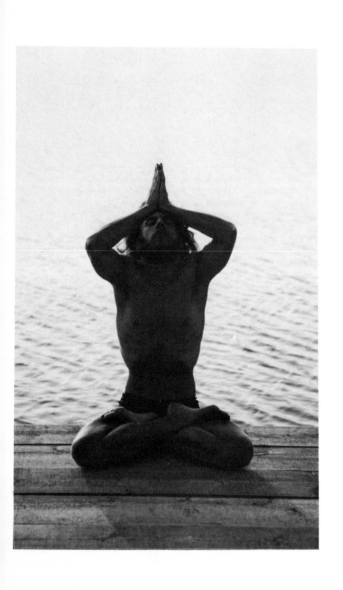

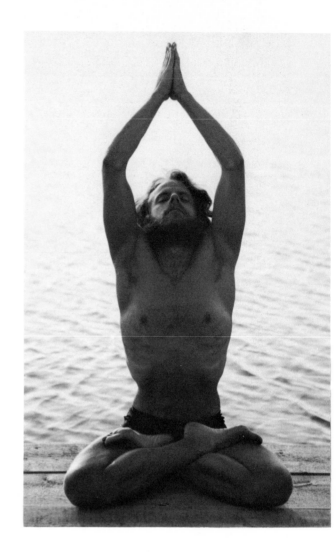

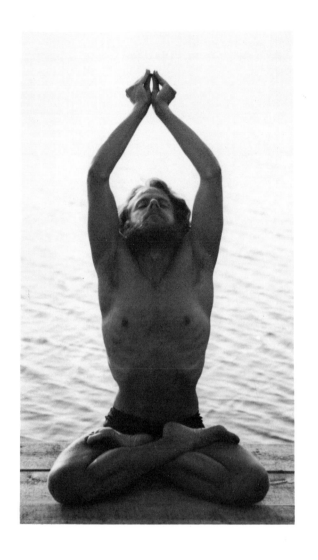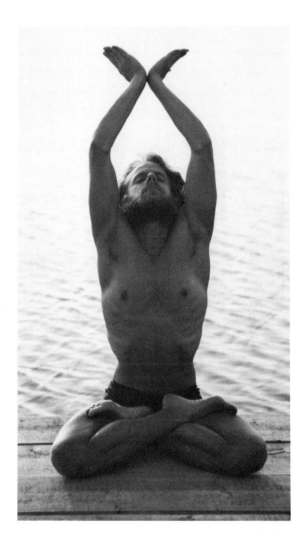

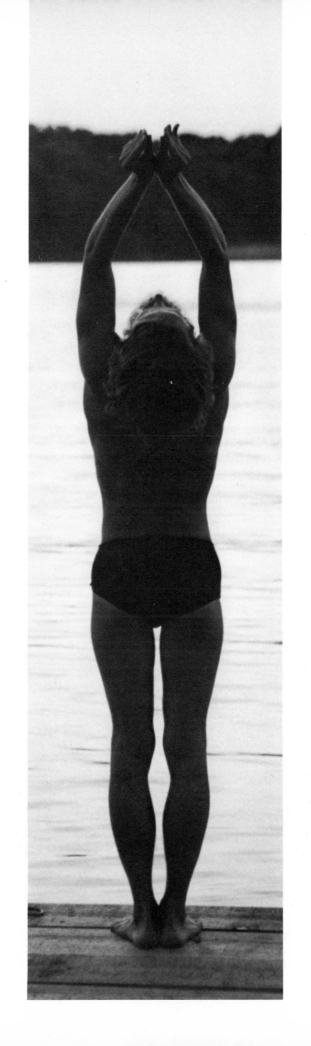

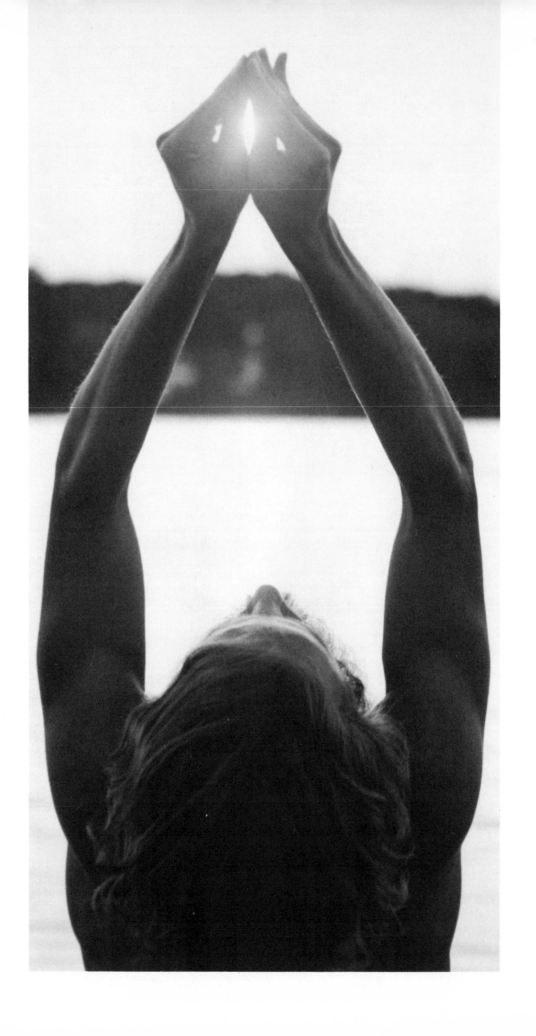

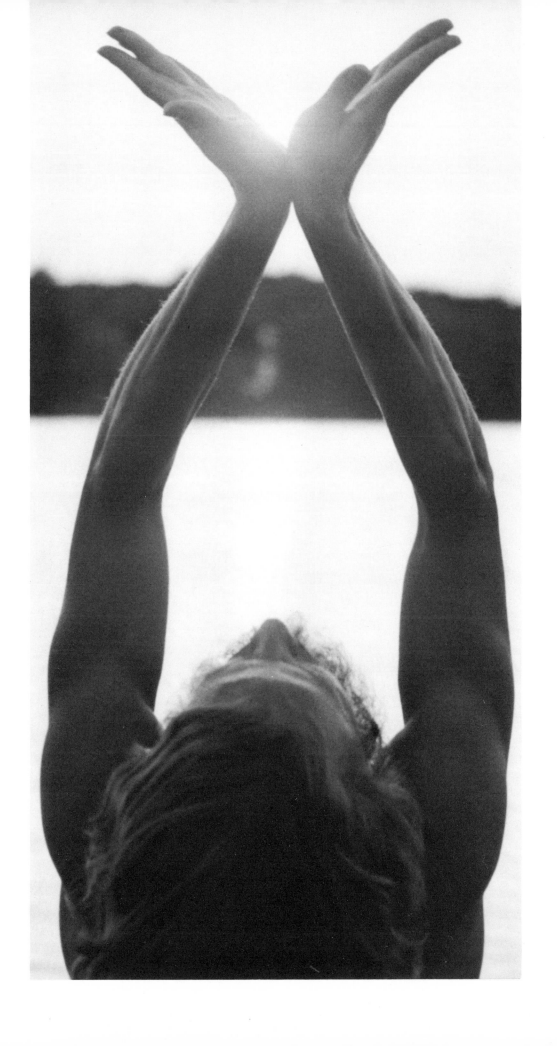

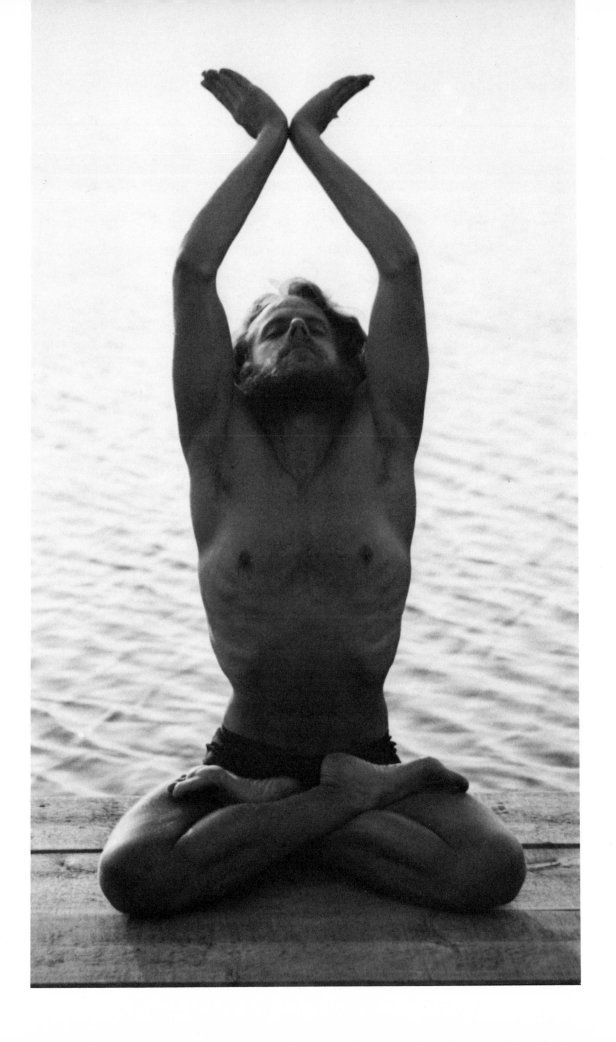

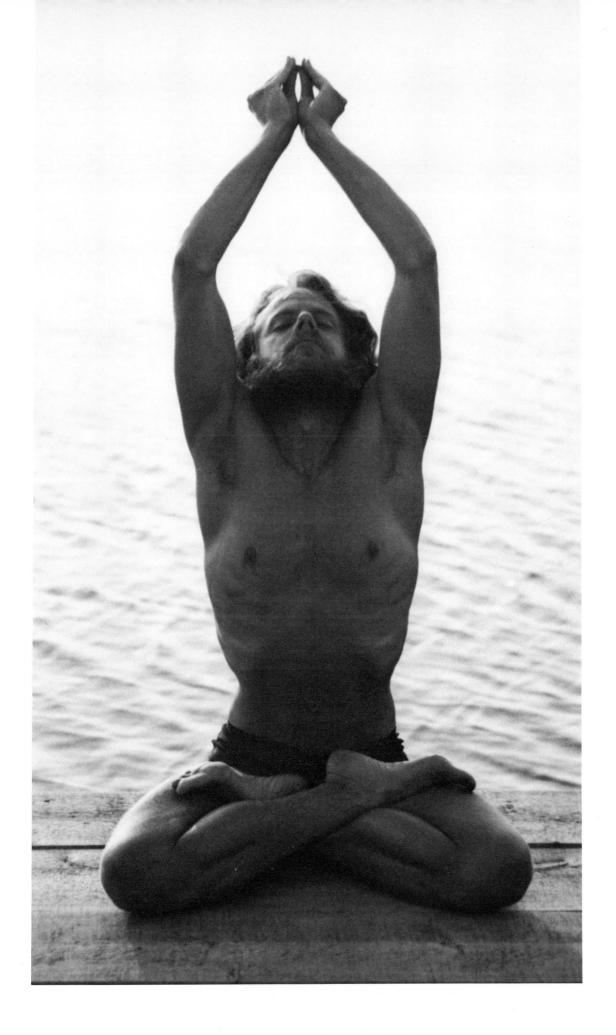

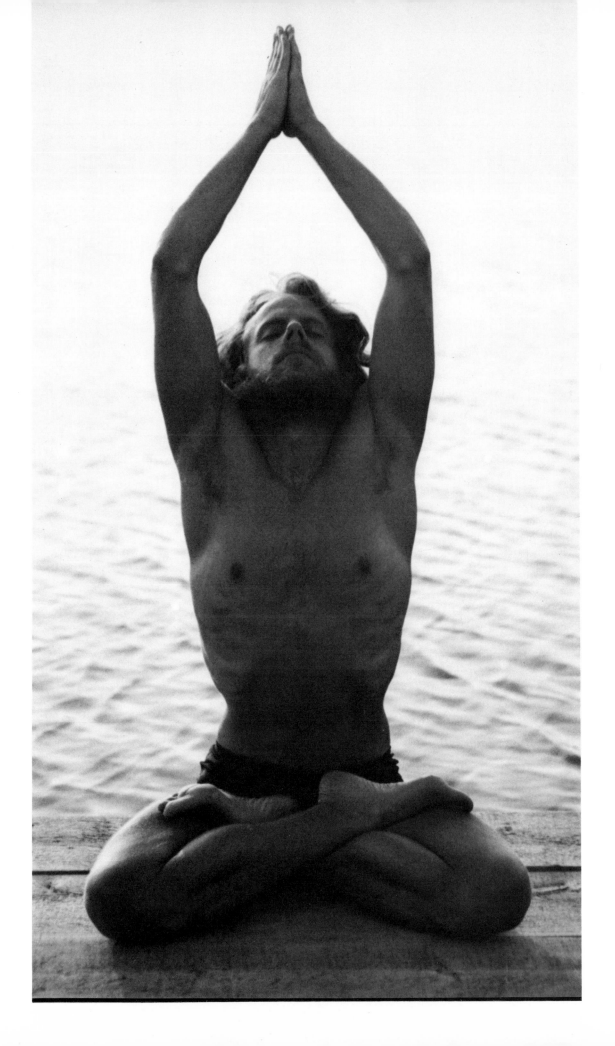

A FINE RESTRAINT JOINS

      FLASHING SUN INTO DARK

      CLEAR MOON.

A SOUND STRIKES

      LIGHT INTO FORM,

      BREATH INTO BODY,

SIFTING BACK AND FORTH

      THE SHINING AIR.

WATERS, STILLED INTO A BREATHING RIPPLE,

      FIND THEIR CUP.

QUIETLY, SIMPLY,

      YOU FIND PLACE.

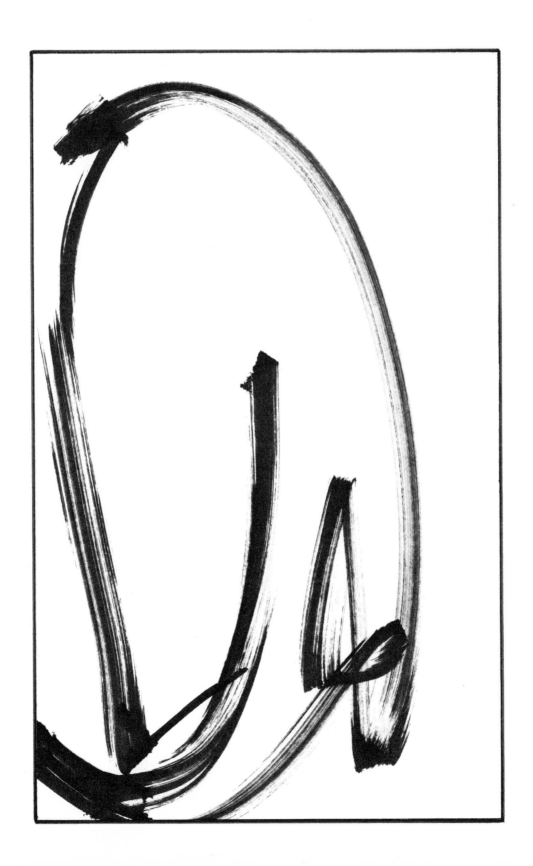

HATHAYOGA ORIGINATED AS *TANTRA*—

A REFORMATIONAL DEVELOPMENT OF YOGA WHICH

EXPANDED *VEDĀNTA* ASCETICISM INTO FULL AND COMPLETE

INVOLVEMENT WITH THE WORLD.

FIRMLY REJECTING EMPTY SPECULATION IN FAVOR

OF SIMPLE DAILY PRACTICE, IT BECAME A LIBERATION OF

SHEER ENTHRALLMENT,

AN ECSTASY OF PLACE SPUN INTO WEAVING ARCS

OF UNIVERSAL VIBRATION.

THIS BOOK IS A VISUAL MEDITATION, OR *YANTRA,* OF

HATHAYOGA. ITS TEXT HAS THE HIGHLY CONCISE PERSONAL

FORM OF TANTRA *VACANA* POETRY, WHILE ITS PHOTOGRAPHS

SHAPE MEDITATION USING THE BEST OF ALL YANTRAS,

THE HUMAN BODY. ITS CULTURAL BACKGROUND MAY BE FOUND

IN THE FOLLOWING PUBLICATIONS:

ELIADE, MIRCEA, *YOGA, IMMORTALITY AND FREEDOM,*
       BOLLINGEN SERIES LVI, PRINCETON UNIVERSITY PRESS,
       PRINCETON, NEW JERSEY, 1958, 1969.

     —TANTRA, PRESENTED PHILOSOPHICALLY IN CHAPTER VI,
     "YOGA AND TANTRISM," PP. 200-273.

RAMANUJAN, A. K. (EDITOR), *SPEAKING OF SIVA,*
       PENGUIN BOOKS, BALTIMORE, MARYLAND, 1973.

     —TANTRA, PRESENTED AS VACANA POETRY.

RAWSON, PHILIP, *THE ART OF TANTRA,* NEW YORK GRAPHIC
       SOCIETY, GREENWICH, CONNECTICUT, 1973.

     —TANTRA, PRESENTED AS VISUAL ART.

ZIMMER, HEINRICH, *MYTHS AND SYMBOLS IN INDIAN ART
       AND CIVILIZATION,* BOLLINGEN SERIES VI (1946),
       PRINCETON UNIVERSITY PRESS, PRINCETON, NEW JERSEY, 1972.

     —TANTRA, PRESENTED MYTHOLOGICALLY IN CHAPTER IV,
     "THE COSMIC DELIGHT OF SIVA", PP. 123-188,
     AND CHAPTER V, "THE GODDESS," PP. 189-216.

THE AUTHOR, W. A. COMPTON, BESIDES TEACHING
HATHAYOGA AT HARVARD UNIVERSITY, IS ALSO
INVOLVED WITH ART AS A FORM OF MEDITATION.
HE BEGAN THIS BOOK IN THE SUMMER OF 1970,
RECEIVING INVALUABLE ASSISTANCE FROM STEVEN
KATONA, WHO HANDLED THE CAMERA, AND FROM
SUSAN LERNER, WHO GAVE HER CALM PRESENCE
AND CRITICAL SUPPORT. IT IS PRESENTED TO THEM
WITH WARMEST THANKS, AND OFFERED FOR PUB-
LICATION IN THE FALL OF 1973.

THE DRAWING—A SINGLE STROKE ENCOMPASSING
SEVEN ARTICULATIONS—IS A YANTRA OF *OM*, THE
MOST BASIC *MANTRA,* OR SOUND MEDITATION OF
HATHAYOGA.

74 75 76 77 78 79 80   12 11 10 9 8 7 6 5 4 3 2 1